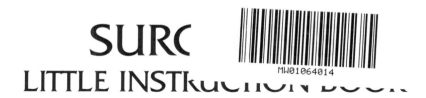

SURG
LITTLE INSTRUCTION BOOK

Daniel James Waters, D.O.

Foreword by Floyd D. Loop, M.D.

Quality Medical Publishing, Inc.

ST. LOUIS, MISSOURI
1998

Printed in the United States of America

Quality Medical Publishing, Inc.
11970 Borman Drive, Suite 222
St. Louis, Missouri 63146
Telephone: 1-800-348-7808
Web site: http://www.qmp.com

ISBN   1-57626-082-8

QMP/VGR/VGR   5 4 3 2 1

For my wife, Pam,
and my children Jessica, Michael, and John

FOREWORD

It's no surprise that Dr. Dan Waters' first book, *A Heart Surgeon's Little Instruction Book,* was a success. Packed with practical axioms from an accomplished surgeon, it is a book to be read easily, shared with friends, and confidently given to colleagues. Now Dr. Waters follows up his initial success with this new volume, *A Surgeon's Little Instruction Book.* We all know how difficult it is to hit a home run in two successive times at bat, but Dr. Waters has done just that.

A Surgeon's Little Instruction Book gives us yet more priceless wisdom, compressed into neat epigrams. The literature of medicine offers no more pleasurable collection of know-how, wisecracks, and well-honed reflections on everything from ethics to economics—much of it original.

The best surgeons don't forget their mistakes, and Dr. Waters' wisdom is clear-eyed and clearly hard-won. There is something here for everyone: the experienced surgeon, nonsurgical specialist, resident, or even layperson looking for insight into the surgical profession.

If you are fortunate enough to have both of Dr. Waters' books, you will find them excellent companions throughout your career. They give you insight into the present, shed new light on the past, and may leave you better prepared for your next case.

Floyd D. Loop, M.D.
Chief Executive Officer
Chairman, Board of Governors
The Cleveland Clinic Foundation
Cleveland, Ohio

ACKNOWLEDGMENTS

Although the individual "instructions" are uncredited, they represent the contributions of many people. My thanks to the surgeons and staff at The Cleveland Clinic Foundation, my wonderful team at North Iowa Mercy Health Center, and to the staff at Quality Medical Publishing. Special thanks to those individuals who took the time to submit their favorite bits of advice for inclusion in this volume:

Guillermo Escobard Aldasoro, M.D.
John Anderson, M.D.
H. Hunt Batjer, M.D.
David E. Beck, M.D.
Burt Brent, M.D.
Sterling Bunnell, M.D.
Allan Callow, M.D.
James Cox, M.D.
Susanne Curn de Escobar, M.D.
Adrian Flatt, M.D.
Hyman Gaylis, M.D.
Philip Glick, M.D.
Philip Gordon, M.D.
James C. Grotting, M.D.

Jonathan Hill, M.D.
Ian T. Jackson, M.D.
Paul MacGregor, D.O.
Keith Naunheim, M.D.
Jeffrey Peters, M.D.
Kendall Reed, D.O.
Kevin Rier, M.D.
Peter Schneider, M.D.
Arthur Smith, M.D.
Lee E. Smith, M.D.
Patti Lynn Trapp, R.N.
Charles W. Van Way, M.D.
Frank Veith, M.D.
Lewis Williams, M.D.

To anyone inadvertently omitted, my sincere apologies.

INTRODUCTION

"Wit is the only wall between us and the dark."

This quote from the American poet and scholar Mark Van Doren perhaps best sums up the genesis of this volume of surgical "wisdom," a follow-up to *A Heart Surgeon's Little Instruction Book.* The enthusiastic response to this previous collection confirmed a long-standing suspicion that there is a wellspring of useful surgical information that rarely sees the printed page. While cardiac surgery certainly has its share of helpful aphorisms, other specialties have their own unique funds as well. In an effort to expand the scope of this book, notable individuals in several surgical disciplines have helped cull their favorite bits of advice. Their contributions range from pointers on the technical aspects of performing a particular operation to the more intuitive arts of dealing with patients, families, and colleagues. But they all share a common theme—that all of us have something to teach and, perhaps more important, something to learn from one another and from those individuals with whose care we are entrusted. I hope that each reader will find in these pages something to think about, something to smile about, and something to remember and pass on.

Daniel J. Waters, D.O.
May 1998

CONTENTS

Preoperative Contemplations

"To be prepared for war is one of the most effectual means of preserving peace."

George Washington

"Conference maketh a ready man."

Francis Bacon

1. Start each case with a clear conscience and an empty bladder.

2. Always do a rectal exam as part of any abdominal examination. If you don't put your finger in it, you may put your foot in it.

3. Remember that there is a fundamental difference between seeing a disease and seeing a *picture* of a disease.

4. The most important part of a surgical consultation is the discussion with the patient.

5. Most surgeons know who to operate on; really good ones know who *not* to operate on.

6. Base your clinical decisions on science, not advertising.

7. Never offer a patient an operation you wouldn't have performed on yourself if you needed it.

8. If you are unhappy with the quality of a diagnostic study, your patient deserves to have it repeated.

9. A preoperative consultation should be performed with at least as much care as the operation itself.

10. Adopt and adhere to your institution's "Appropriateness Criteria" for your surgical specialty.

11. Never commit to operating on a patient without actually seeing him or her.

12. Treat patients, not pictures!

13. Just because you can justify an operation doesn't necessarily mean you should perform it.

14. There is no such thing as too much documentation.

15. Almost every decision ultimately boils down to *risk* and *benefit*.

16. When faced with the choice between *slim* and *none,* most patients will choose slim.

17. A preoperative risk-stratification system should be used when possible; the results may surprise you.

18. Combined operations deserve careful deliberation.

19. "Ornery" patients tend to live longer.

20. In cardiac surgery:
You *have* to do emergencies.
You *have* to do redos.
You *don't have* to do emergency redos.

21. If you don't feel good about performing an operation, don't do it.

22. Preoperative duplex mapping of venous conduits can help avoid many an unpleasant surprise.

23. When pressured to accept a difficult case, never underestimate the bravery of a noncombatant.

24. If you worry about things that *might* happen, a lot of the things you worry about *won't* happen.

25. In patients with poor left ventricular function, a preoperative period of intra-aortic balloon counterpulsation can turn a climb into a walk.

26. Actively include the patient's spouse in the discussion of a proposed operation.

27. In reoperations, always take the time to read closely the previous operative note. Much information is contained not only *in* but also *between* the lines.

28. Never discourage a patient who wants a second opinion.

29. Investigate carotid bruits *before* a cardiac operation.

30. In younger patients undergoing revascularization procedures, discuss the possibility of future interventions despite the success of the initial operation.

31. If at all possible, get the operative consent signed yourself.

32. Make it a point to listen for subclavian bruits in any patient who will be receiving an internal thoracic artery graft.

33. Don't be *afraid* to perform a new procedure, just be *prepared.*

34. Technology is sometimes more advanced than our ability to apply it properly.

35. In patients with lung disease, a few days of *preparation* can often save a few weeks of *ventilation*.

36. Know your limitations, preferably ahead of time.

37. Always check the level of magnification used for angiography; the actual vessels may well be smaller than they appear.

38. If a preoperative patient tells you that he or she is going to die, immediately cancel the operation.

39. Never be afraid to turn down a bad case.

40. When the chances of success are slim and none, make sure "slim" isn't out of town.

41. If the septal perforators are visualized, a totally occluded left anterior descending coronary artery is usually graftable.

42. Don't lose sight of the fact that treatment may carry more risk than the underlying disease in some patients.

43. The three most important determinants of surgical outcomes are:
1. Patient selection!
2. Patient selection!
3. Patient selection!

44. If your only tool is a hammer, everything tends to look like a nail.

Operative Techniques and Technology

"They detest the calm who know the storm."

Dorothy Parker

"I am the wound and the knife."

Charles Baudelaire

45. The pancreas is like a skunk—you either have to kill it or leave it alone.

46. Everyone looks older covered in Betadine.

47. Remember that opening and closing are also included in the operative time.

48. Be wary of new technology looking for a job.

49. A midline laparotomy is about as stressful as a haircut.

50. Some patients are not candidates for a haircut.

51. Even if you cut it three times, it will still be too short.

52. Never guess when you can *know.*

53. When closing a scrotal incision, remember that it is hard to make it look any worse!

54. Antibiotics cannot compensate for poor technique.

55. If you stay in the midline, you won't hurt anything.

56. Unless you're doing cardiac surgery, when in doubt, take it out.

57. Treat brain tissue with gentleness, respect, and most of all wonder.

58. If you feel the need to talk during a neurosurgical procedure . . . don't!

59. Keep the neuro OR quiet; it is not a train station.

60. Wear loupes when necessary.

61. Remember:
C3, 4, and 5 keep the diaphragm alive.
But S2, 3, and 4 keep the penis off the floor!

62. Some assistants cannot help you without leaving the room.

63. Making a procedure more complex doesn't necessarily make it better.

64. If you continue to fight, an arteriovenous malformation will ultimately fatigue.

65. The five words most commonly associated with a reoperation for bleeding are, *"I think that will stop."*

66. Although a wound heals from side to side and not from end to end, a smaller hole is usually a better hole.

67. The difference between cardiac surgery and invasive cardiology is the difference between real life and TV.

68. An assistant who can't *see* the problem can rarely *help* with the solution.

69. Large-caliber venous conduits have to be measured precisely as they are likely to kink if cut too long.

70. No flow, no leak.

71. Some operations are difficult even if you are doing them correctly.

72. In cardiac operations, remember that almost every heart looks good at 5 liters.

73. Don't throw instruments.

74. If you *must* throw something, make it something disposable.

75. Every distal anastomosis should be a little Rembrandt.

76. It is the technique not the forceps that needs to be atraumatic.

77. Deliver retrograde cerebral perfusion during circulatory arrest.

78. Know at least two alternative sites for arterial cannulation for cardiopulmonary bypass.

79. Surgical loupes magnify your field, not necessarily your ability.

80. If some things in surgery don't scare you, they should.

81. Freshen the end of a vein graft *with a scalpel* just prior to anastomosing it.

82. Keep an arterial pedicle moist with a vasodilator solution *during as well as after* its procurement.

83. Clip side branches on venous conduits so that they are perfectly flush with the lumen.

84. When a stitch breaks, it is less often the fault of the suture than the jerk at the end.

85. Speed in operating is nothing more than economy of movement.

86. You are in a great specialty if hemostasis can often be achieved by the application of little white sponges.

87. The pump-oxygenator is not a "resurrection machine."

88. If you only do routine cases, eventually *they* will seem difficult.

89. The surgeon should control access to cardio-pulmonary bypass technology.

90. After cardiopulmonary bypass, give a "test dose" of protamine before decannulating.

91. Every five years a new procedure threatens to do away with conventional coronary bypass surgery. This will continue until you retire.

92. Be suspicious of procedures that are "hyped" to the general public before they are proved to be advantageous or beneficial.

93. Many cardiac surgeons would change their spouse before they would change their aortic cannula.

94. In reoperations, the appearance of the old scar can sometimes indicate the extent of adhesions.

95. Don't ask your institution to purchase new technology just because "it's cool."

96. In some specialties, angioplasty is the gift that just keeps on giving.

97. A surgeon who doesn't know the name of an instrument may not be qualified to use it.

98. No procedure should be called minimally invasive if more than four separate incisions are required.

99. In cardiac reoperation, the initial identification of the pericardial plane is the single most important technical maneuver.

100. It is always less stressful to take someone else's patient back to the operating room for bleeding.

101. Some ideas that were bad before may yet be bad ideas again.

102. Femoral cannulation for cardiopulmonary bypass is neither ubiquitous nor assuredly benign.

103. Pulmonary disease is the most common predictor of sternotomy problems.

104. Limited incisions can also mean limited options.

105. In younger patients, do the little things that make reoperation easier for the next surgeon—It might be *you!*

106. Use electrocautery to "spot weld" the tissue, not to vaporize it.

107. The newer antithrombotics can promote bleeding that is all but unstoppable; check to see if a patient has been treated with one of them.

108. When operating on the carotid artery, remember, don't "craque the plaque."

109. Never buy a piece of equipment that requires a salesman to come into the OR to show you how to use it.

110. An ophthalmologic scalpel is superb for performing a coronary arteriotomy.

111. In surgical advances, instrumentation often lags behind imagination.

112. Leaving a bad vessel ungrafted may cause less morbidity than trying to endarterectomize it.

113. Dry up your patients with the same meticulousness whether you are on call or not.

114. In isolated valve operations, always prep the legs as well as the chest.

115. If blood hits the light, a named vessel has been transected.

116. If you operate with magnification, peripheral *hearing* is more important than peripheral *vision*.

117. It is not the size of your cannula, but its performance that counts.

118. Avoid long-duration "burns" with the electrocautery; the ambient heat generated can be insidious and damaging.

119. If the tip of the cautery pen will fit into the end of a vessel, that vessel *must* be ligated.

120. The three most common causes of hypotension following esophageal resection are hypovolemia, hypovolemia, and hypovolemia!

121. The success of many "less invasive" procedures depends as much on the anesthesia team as it does on the surgeon.

122. Be circumspect when you dismiss new ideas or new technology.

123. Always check your sutures—there are the "haves" and the "have knots."

124. Momentarily discontinue balloon counterpulsation when cannulating or decannulating the aorta.

125. In coronary revascularization, judging graft length is more art than science.

126. The request to "raise the table" should always be prefaced with "watch the feet."

127. After median sternotomy, the pneumothorax on POD 1 comes not from the hole that is in the pleura but from the one that *isn't.*

128. Always consider a pulmonary artery catheter as a source of unexplained ventricular dysrhythmias after surgery.

129. In cardiac reoperation, "cheat" a little to the right side when reopening the sternum; many a patent internal thoracic artery graft has been avoided in this manner.

130. If you have an idea that retention sutures are needed, they probably are.

131. Remember that in esophageal surgery it ain't over till the fat lady swallows.

132. Epicardial pacing wires usually prevent more morbidity than they ever cause.

133. Always prep and drape too large a field; the one time you don't is the one time you'll wish you had.

134. The surgeon should always be the person who directs separation from cardiopulmonary bypass.

135. Placing an open sternal spreader before using an internal mammary artery retractor can help reduce the "left shift" of the chest wall in median sternotomy.

136. There is no "cone of silence" at the OR table. Be circumspect in your cross-table discussions.

137. Hemostasis is often better in the dark.

138. Keep the OR temperature in mind during each phase of a long operation.

139. Remember that all arterial conduits are not created equal.

140. Placing stitches too close together in a vessel can cause them to act like perforations in paper and can actually weaken an anastomosis.

141. Individually ligating the thymic branches of the innominate vein can significantly lessen tension placed on it during median sternotomy.

142. If you can't see it, you can't sew it.

143. Don't grasp the right atrial wall with forceps outside of the confines of a pursestring or suture line.

144. In patients with ventricular failure, don't get fooled into operating on "situational" mitral regurgitation.

145. Never forget that even minor procedures can have major complications.

146. The aggregate sum of incision lengths for a procedure to be called "minimally invasive" should be less than the length of the standard incision.

147. The lesser saphenous veins can be harvested with the patient in the supine position, but more grunting is required.

148. Controlled blood pressure at the time of incision is worth waiting for.

149. Keep the ends of epicardial pacing wires well away from grafts, especially on the right.

150. Minimalism, like its artistic counterpart, is not for everyone.

151. In vascular reoperations, be wary of distal hypoperfusion when replacing a large-caliber conduit with a smaller one.

152. Never dismiss a new technology out of hand. Its ultimate use and value can often be much different from its initial application.

153. In incisions, as in other aspects of anatomy, it is always debatable as to whether size is important.

154. Anesthetic management should be an *interactive* process.

155. New technologies often need time to "mature" before they can be widely or *wisely* applied.

156. After a certain point in heparin reversal, more protamine can mean more bleeding.

157. Place transthoracic defibrillator patches on all patients undergoing cardiac reoperation.

158. Audible bleeding is usually a poor prognostic sign.

159. It is important but often difficult to differentiate between fads, innovations, and true breakthroughs in surgical procedures.

160. Keep a valvulotome in your vascular instrument set; some veins are better conduits in the nonreversed position.

161. Never tell a resident who is tying a knot, "Whatever you do, don't break it."

162. In carotid surgery, shunts are for wimps.

163. In carotid surgery, wimps often have better outcomes.

164. Use caution when using procoagulants in cases where circulatory arrest is planned.

165. Preservation of the vascular endothelium in revascularization conduits cannot be emphasized enough.

166. In valve replacement, use the enhanced exposure as you place the annular stitches to "fine-tune" your debridement.

167. Your fingertips are still the most important "instrument" you have.

168. Electronic atrioventricular pacing can sometimes be the culprit when encountering unexpected difficulty in weaning a patient from cardiopulmonary bypass.

169. If at all possible, avoid reopening the sternum anywhere but in the operating room.

170. In cardiac reoperation, the road to hell is paved with felt pledgets.

171. In routine cardiac cases, topical cooling may carry more risk than benefit.

172. In cases of severe coagulopathy, sometimes you just have to close and treat the deficiencies, knowing that you will probably go back in later.

173. Always keep a forceps in one hand when assisting—it is never wise to be unarmed during battle.

174. Avoid out-of-body experiences while assisting the staff surgeon.

175. An acceptable assistant should breathe at least four times a minute.

176. Don't clip or clamp atherosclerotic grafts as this may embolize the distal vessel with debris.

177. In reoperation in younger cardiac patients, avoid dissecting the space between the aorta and the pulmonary artery.

178. Avoid pressurizing a vascular conduit above systemic levels; intimal damage is likely.

179. Age should only be one factor in the decision to utilize an arterial conduit for coronary revascularization.

180. Don't panic—even when it is obviously the most rational thing to do.

181. Keep in mind that a "new" operation may turn out to be like disco dancing—in two years you'll be bragging that you *didn't* do it.

Postoperative Considerations

"O' polished perturbation! Golden care!
That keep'st the ports of slumber open wide
To many a watchful night!"

William Shakespeare
Henry IV

". . . So many incidents, so many details."

Constantine Peter Cavafy

182. In a patient who is doing well, don't just do something—Stand there!

183. After a difficult case that goes well, avoid "premature rejoicing"—disaster almost always ensues.

184. A good operation deserves a good operative note and dictation.

185. Never relinquish the care of your postoperative patients to anyone but your partners.

186. If the pupils remain small, the soul usually cannot escape.

187. Many postoperative problems have their roots in the OR.

188. Inotropes after cardiopulmonary bypass are like catapults on aircraft carriers. They won't keep you flying, but they can get you airborne.

189. Blood conservation is great, but don't underestimate the subtle impact of anemia on the patient's recovery.

190. Be cautious in the use of procoagulants after a revascularization procedure; a little oozing is preferable to a clotted graft.

191. Even in small doses, psychotropic medications can have profound effects on the elderly postoperative patient.

192. Cure postoperative atrial fibrillation and the world will beat a path to your door.

193. Successful postoperative care is dependent on meticulous attention to detail. So check everything. Twice!

194. Design and practice a "lifeboat drill" with your ICU nurses in the event of sudden and exsanguinating postoperative hemorrhage.

195. The number of restraints placed on a patient is directly proportional to his or her likelihood to escape them.

196. Unexplained restlessness in a postoperative cardiac patient can be a subtle sign of delayed tamponade.

197. In the immediate postoperative period, to pee is to live.

198. Make sure *someone* is following a young patient's lipid profile after revascularization surgery.

199. A change of location is a common time for patients to suffer a complication.

200. When abscess is a consideration, it is usually better to "look and see" than it is to "wait and see."

201. Never walk by the ICU without stopping to see your patients.

202. If you think about intubating a patient, you should probably do it; one of the most common mistakes is to intubate too late.

203. Dictate your operative note as soon after surgery as possible.

204. See your immediate postoperative patients *just once more* before leaving the hospital.

205. In a patient who is doing well, keep in mind the primary rule of postoperative management—Don't mess with success!

Residents, Staff, and Colleagues

"Who shall decide when doctors disagree?"

Alexander Pope

"Don't be humble; you're not that great."

Golda Meir

206. Residents are like Persian carpets—trod upon daily and beaten once a year.

207. Surgical interns are easy to maintain as there are usually no moving parts.

208. When assisting, at least pretend you are going to help.

209. Remind your residents that while conferences may not be mandatory, neither is program graduation.

210. Aspire to the level of the surgeons who trained you.

211. Treat your colleagues as partners and your partners as colleagues.

212. Don't be harder on your team than you are on yourself.

213. Don't shoot the anesthesiologists; they are doing the best they can.

214. Weather the slings and arrows of outrageous referring physicians with as much humor as possible.

215. Always state the facts clearly to the attending surgeon; it is better to be found wrong than dishonest.

216. Be wary of a colleague who is duplicitous in his or her personal life; a white coat may hide stripes but it will rarely change them.

217. Beware the physician who is seldom right but never in doubt.

218. You'll understand the true value of a good perfusionist only after you've had a bad one.

219. Don't overlook the contribution that your secretary makes to the success of your practice.

220. Advice is the currency exchanged between surgeons.

221. In general, the most aggressive cardiac surgeons are usually cardiologists.

222. When on call, remember that a surprised staff surgeon is an *unhappy* staff surgeon.

223. Breathe at least four times a minute.

224. Referrals should not be looked upon as gifts or favors, but rather as entrusted decisions about the welfare of fellow human beings.

225. You don't train at an institution in order to bestow the gift of *your* insight on the staff.

226. Realize that your team watches *everything* you do.

227. Care for your partners' patients with the same enthusiasm you do for your own.

228. Remember that part of your responsibility as a resident is to assume blame for things that are not your fault.

229. Apologize for bad behavior in the OR—the sooner, the better.

230. Always be nice to the hospital switchboard operators.

231. *NEVER* tell one staff surgeon how another staff surgeon "does it."

232. Be wary of colleagues who are more familiar with their billings than they are with their results.

233. Don't blame the nurses for your mistakes.

234. Large institutions are rife with "palace intrigue"—*Trust no one.*

235. Work *with* referring doctors, never *for* them.

236. Don't depend on anyone else to do your work for you.

237. Your younger partners should be able to teach you as well as learn from you.

238. Never demean a colleague in front of a patient or family member; it makes you both look bad.

239. Learn to recognize the difference between colleagues who are doctors and those who are entrepreneurs with medical degrees.

240. Call your consultants *personally* when requesting their services.

241. Your surgical team notices the color of your socks—just imagine what *else* they notice.

242. Never forget that until you are out of training, they are not *your* patients.

243. Acknowledge the efforts of the hospital's housekeeping and maintenance workers. Patients look at their work almost as much as yours.

244. Disagree with your partners privately; support them publicly.

245. It is sometimes necessary to remind a referring specialist that the procedure is performed on the *patient* and not on the diagnostic study.

246. Most surgeons think their cases are tougher, sicker, and more complicated than everyone else's.

247. Spending time teaching your ICU nurses is one of the best investments you can make.

248. Be skeptical of colleagues who insist they *never* see a particular complication.

249. Learn quickly to recognize when a referral is just someone wanting his or her problem to become *your* problem.

250. Being a good assistant sometimes entails more work than performing the operation.

251. The drapes should never be an obstacle to good communication with the anesthesia providers.

252. If your nurses or residents are ever *afraid* to call you, you have bigger problems than you realize.

253. If you are "on-line," be wary of pontificating cybersurgeons.

254. Make it a point to remember Nurses' Day and Secretaries' Day.

255. It is almost always more fun to operate with your partners than without them.

256. If you find two colleagues you can really trust, you're twice as lucky as most.

257. Some days referral relations can be the most stressful part of a surgical practice.

258. Always keep in mind that surgery is truly a *team* effort.

259. When checking references of a prospective partner, make it a point to talk to the OR and ICU nurses as well. The information you get may be very illuminating.

260. Never send a resident or secretary to do your birthday or Christmas shopping.

261. If most nonsurgical interventionalists could see and feel the vessels they are manipulating, they would run screaming into the night.

262. Protect your assistants and surgical team members from blood exposure just as you would yourself.

263. Despite the assumptions of some referring specialists, saphenous veins do not come standard out of a box.

264. No one is ever exactly who they seem during a job interview.

265. A watched interventionalist never dilates.

266. *Tell* the resident whether to cut the suture too long or too short—it will save time.

267. On night duty all residents are promoted one year.

268. Never, but never, antagonize the head nurse in the OR.

269. Your team makes you look better than you probably are.

270. As a resident, remember that it is not time to be creative after the staff surgeon leaves the room.

271. Don't date an OR nurse unless you intend to marry one.

272. Sooner or later you have to stand up for what's right, even if it means losing a referral.

273. A resident called for a problem with a patient should *always go see the patient.*

274. Try to remember that the members of your team have lives, too.

275. As a senior resident, it is often quicker and more efficient to do a task yourself than to delegate it to the person one step below in the hierarchy.

276. A resident who mismanages a bad situation or complication should be admonished; a resident who conceals a bad situation should be dismissed.

277. Thank your team at the end of each case, particularly after a difficult one.

278. You will most often be forgiven fits of pique as long as you don't personalize them.

279. Invite your referring physicians to observe during surgery.

280. Never expect a nonsurgeon to *really* understand what goes into getting a patient through an operation.

281. When operating with senior staff always remember that the phrase, "Let me show you a little trick," is often followed by the phrase, "Oh my God! Suture!"

282. The general difference between surgical residents and canine excreta is that staff surgeons usually don't go out of their way to step on the latter.

283. In the event of a complication, the resident closest to the bed is assigned the blame.

THE SURGICAL ASSISTANT'S PHRASEBOOK
(with translations)

"I'm not sure Dr. X would do it quite that way."
Translation: *The staff surgeon will fire you if he sees this.*

"You're the best, sir (or ma'am)."
Translation: *You're an idiot.*

"That's certainly innovative."
Translation: *It's the stupidest idea I have ever heard.*

"Would you mind if I made a suggestion?"
Translation: *Do it this way or I'll have to hurt you.*

"Oh, you certainly are brave."
Translation: *What in the world are you doing?*

"Do you think you want to let the staff surgeon know about this?"
Translation: *I'm not getting fired for something you did.*

"Let me see if I can expose that better for you."
Translation: *Cut right here.*

THE SURGICAL ASSISTANT'S PHRASEBOOK—cont'd

"Sorry."
Translation: *Your operating is interfering with my assisting.*

"What's for lunch today?"
Translation: *This case is taking too damn long.*

"I'm here to help you."
Translation: *You're on your own.*

"I'm sure the staff surgeon will understand."
Translation: *Can I have your locker when you're gone?*

"I think you might be getting the hang of this."
Translation: *I can't believe it. You did something right.*

"Excuse me, am I in your way?"
Translation: *Move—you're in my way.*

"Maybe I can get that better from here."
Translation: *Give me that instrument before you hurt someone!*

"I think it's dry enough to close."
Translation: *I'm not on call.*

THE SURGICAL ASSISTANT'S PHRASEBOOK—cont'd

"Maybe we should take one more look around."
Translation: *I am on call.*

"Well, that case didn't go too badly."
Translation: *The Exxon Valdez had a smoother voyage.*

"Let me know if I can help you."
Translation: *Don't ask me to do anything.*

"The anatomy sure wasn't straightforward today."
Translation: *Are you sure you're a doctor?*

"I'm glad to see you're being careful."
Translation: *This case is going to take all day.*

"Help me understand the thinking behind that."
Translation: *Are you out of your mind?*

"Nice job."
Translation: *Unavailable; no record of ever actually being said.*

Publications and Presentations

"I am a galley slave to pen and ink."

Honoré de Balzac

"The great questions of the time are not decided by speeches. . . ."

Otto von Bismarck

284. Never let a published scientific article stand in the way of common sense.

285. Read at least one nonsurgical journal monthly.

286. Attend meetings that have presentations, not advertisements.

287. Understand the following translations:

"In my experience"	One case
"In case after case"	Two cases
"In my series"	Three or four cases

288. If you can't baffle 'em with brilliance, dazzle 'em with data.

289. Statistical data are like swimsuits—encouraging in their revelation, vital in their concealment.

290. Just because something appears in a journal does not necessarily mean it is a good idea.

291. Don't confuse advertising copy with clinical information.

292. Never confuse a meeting with reality.

293. Owning a surgical text does not automatically confer the knowledge contained therein.

294. Don't say "paradigm shift" more than once a year.

295. Even if you're not a frequent contributor, on-line discussion forums can be of great value.

296. The following disclaimer should be shown at the end of all procedural videos:
The operation on the screen was actually more difficult than it appeared!

297. Scientific presentations should not be "infomercials" for products, surgeons, or institutions.

298. Requests for reprints are a sincere form of flattery.

299. At M & M conferences, the ABCs of surgical case defense are: *A*ccuse, *B*lame, and *C*riticize.

300. Motto for scientific meetings: "Abandon all hype ye who enter here."

301. Try your hand at writing a book; you never know!

302. How surgeons at different levels read a scientific article:

First-year resident	Reads entire article
Senior resident	Reads abstract
Chief resident	Reads author location and affiliation for job possibility
Junior staff	Checks authors' names to see what peers are doing
Senior staff	Checks references to see if quoted
Emeritus staff	Doesn't read—published same findings years ago

Business, Politics, and Other Clinical Perils

"So much more businesslike than businessmen. . . ."

Robert Frost

"The door is open but the ride, it ain't free."

Bruce Springsteen

303. There are many doctors who are great and many doctors who are wealthy, but there are few who are both.

304. Completing your medical records in a timely manner is a responsibility, not a favor.

305. Participate in continuous quality improvement programs.

306. Forgive litigious attorneys, but write down their names.

307. If you ever wonder if surgery is really an art, take a look at the number of critics.

308. Beware of "entangling alliances" with equipment and pharmaceutical vendors.

309. Never work for a chairman who doesn't promote his or her staff.

310. The hardest part of putting together a clinical trial is coming up with a catchy acronym for it.

311. Avoid even the appearance of professional conflict of interest.

312. Never assume an administrator knows more about your practice than you do.

313. Treat your technical sales representatives cordially; their jobs are important to them, too.

314. The Seven Deadly Sins in surgical practice
   are:
   1. Greed
   2. Arrogance
   3. Greed
   4. Arrogance
   5. Greed
   6. Arrogance
   7. Greed

315. Be scrupulous in your documentation in and out of the OR.

316. Always read over your dictation before signing it.

317. The need for cost containment is real—Deal with it!

318. Participate in a nationally recognized surgical database.

319. A physician who takes a course and comes back an "executive" should be viewed the same way as an executive who takes a course and returns as a "physician."

320. Retirement planning should begin the day you enter practice.

321. Start funding your children's education as soon as possible.

322. Have a will drawn up—You only *think* you're immortal.

323. Include a certain phrase or description in your operative note if you *never* want to operate on a particular patient again.

324. Document your indications for blood and component usage.

325. Even if you don't practice at an "academic" institution, hold a regular M & M conference.

326. As unappealing as it may seem, you have to become involved with the politics of health care.

327. At some institutions the ABCs of resuscitation are:
*A*ssign *B*lame and *C*over your backside.

328. Everyone in your practice who interacts with the patient is involved in risk management.

329. Document in the record your recommendation to patients that they cease cigarette smoking permanently.

330. Three things are certain: Death, taxes, and more meetings.

331. Maintain diplomatic relations with the local media.

332. A certain amount of paranoia is healthy— Whoever your "they" might be, they *are* out to get you.

333. You need to admit your mistakes; you don't need to advertise them.

334. Never underestimate your competition.

335. You should know the cost of everything you use in the OR.

336. A real progress note should contain more than "As above" and "See below."

337. Malpractice litigation is usually less about right and wrong than it is about moving money around.

338. While it is good to be media savvy, it is more important to be media wary.

339. Most problems in physician partnerships revolve around two things: money and call.

340. If you are on a hospital committee, skip half the meetings. You will get a reputation for being busy and you won't miss anything.

341. A good week is when you have more cases than meetings.

342. Take time to read the nurse's notes; the lawyers certainly will.

343. Make cost containment an ongoing process in your program.

344. Don't use the operative note to pat yourself on the back.

345. Don't be a corporate shill.

346. The definition of a clinical joint venture is when the physician does it and the hospital pays for it.

347. If you think you don't need to know about things like "market share" and "competitive positioning," *you're wrong* (unfortunately)!

348. Look critically at your results; everyone else is.

Patients and Their Families

"Remain sitting at your table and listen."

Franz Kafka

*"Every unhappy family
is unhappy in its own way."*

Leo Tolstoi

349. When a patient is not making progress, don't hesitate to seek another opinion; it may save you the embarrassment of having the patient request one first.

350. You make a lifelong friend when you cure urinary retention.

351. Risk management begins at the bedside.

352. Tell patients that smoking is to atherosclerosis what lighter fluid is to charcoal.

353. A patient who says, "I might sue," in a hospital is like a passenger who says, "I might hijack," on a airplane. It immediately and irrevocably changes everything, and never for the better.

354. Realize that *every* patient has something to teach you.

355. You can't demand that every patient have surgery, but you should demand that every patient have choices.

356. Do what is right for the patient, not the referring physician.

357. "Difficult" patients are often the most loyal and the most grateful.

358. In cardiac surgery, remember that just because you can fix their hearts doesn't mean that you can fix their lives.

359. Once the operation is over, patients do most of the work.

360. When it comes to surgery, physicians should make *recommendations* and patients should make *choices*.

361. Visit your previous patients if they are readmitted to the hospital for any reason.

362. For most cardiac surgical patients, the endotracheal tube is the most unpleasant part of the surgical experience.

363. Tailor the operation to the patient, not the patient to the operation.

364. Remember that all the points on a "learning curve" are real people with real lives.

365. Your biggest responsibility at consultation is to explain things to the patient and family members in terms *they* can understand.

366. Never lose track of who the patient's true "primary" doctor is. His or her input can often be crucial.

367. Clearly understand the difference between what the patient needs and what the patient will "tolerate."

368. Your bedside manner is still your most valuable clinical skill.

369. Pay attention to medical articles in the popular press. These are what the patients and their families read.

370. Most malpractice suits are the result of poor communication between physicians and patients or families.

371. Always knock before you enter an exam room and say goodbye when you leave.

372. The operation isn't over until you have talked with the family.

373. Call to check on the patient the day after discharge.

374. Never blame a patient for his or her disease.

375. Make it a point not to talk to a patient's family with blood on your cap, mask, scrubs, or shoe covers.

376. Explain everything to a family twice in simple phrases; then ask if they have any questions.

377. Be honest with patients about whether a procedure is curative or merely palliative.

378. Find something nice to say about the patient's personal physician.

379. Always speak to *someone* in the patient's family before an operation.

380. The decision about whether an operation is the "right" thing to do is always the patient's decision to make.

381. Never make promises about results or outcomes.

382. On a crowded ward, never leave without a kind word, reassurance, or explanation to the patient.

383. For a family in a surgical waiting room, time moves very slowly; send word from the OR about every hour, especially during long or high-risk operations.

384. When speaking to a large group of family members after surgery, try to look at each person at some time during the discussion.

385. When visiting with patients or families, sit down as if you had all day, even when you don't.

386. The key to the care of patients is caring for your patients.

387. Identify the family member who is closest to the patient—spouse, child, sibling, or whoever—and involve that person in your discussion of the proposed operation.

388. More than anything else, patients and families want honesty and straightforwardness from their surgeon, even in the worst situations.

389. Elderly patients are like potato chips—
if handled roughly, they will crumble.

390. Introduce yourself to patients and family
members at each visit. You're not *that* important.

391. When complications occur, be straightforward
and prompt in informing patients and families.

392. Remember that while the patient may think you're wonderful, the family usually isn't so sure.

393. Don't rush to put nasogastric feeding tubes in elderly patients—the physiologic benefit can sometimes be outweighed by the negative psychological impact.

394. Don't avoid the family of a patient who is not doing well.

395. When it stops being about the patient and starts being about the procedure, it's time to take a hard look at what you're doing.

Surgical Reflections

"It is not wisdom to be only wise. . . ."

George Santayana

"Mistakes are always paid for
in casualties. . . ."

Dwight D. Eisenhower

396. Of course you would be a great surgeon, if *only* you had better assistants.

397. In any operation, no matter how routine, always have a "plan B."

398. Remember that some of the best surgical advice never makes it into print.

399. Visit the institution that trained you every few years—what you hold sacred may well have changed.

400. There is a fine line between "pushing the envelope" and human experimentation.

401. It is better to discover a small innovation that *all* surgeons can use.

402. Most "revolutions" in surgery are actually just civil disturbances.

403. You're only as good as your last case.

404. Even famous surgeons put on their scrub pants one leg at a time.

405. In terms of patient expectations, heart surgery is a victim of its own success.

406. Vascular patients with lesions that are easy to fix usually don't need any interventional treatment.

407. Don't underestimate the power of media influence on the "science" of clinical practice.

408. *In vivo veritas.*

409. Remember that there are "land mines" in even the most routine cases.

410. All bleeding stops eventually.

411. Call it what you will, any bleeding that occurs after an operation is "surgical bleeding."

412. Heart surgeons have it easier than colon surgeons—at least blood clots!

413. There are just some cases where *everything* is difficult.

414. Never forget what it was like to be a resident.

415. You should know two ways to do just about everything.

416. Remember "Ocham's scalpel"—The simplest operation is usually the best.

417. The biggest part of doing a difficult operation is thinking that you *can*.

418. The operations for ASD and PDA are merely opportunities for the congenital heart surgeon to look bad.

419. When faced with the choice between brilliance and common sense, choose common sense every time.

420. Self-congratulation before the end of a difficult case almost always portends disaster.

421. Beware any part of an operation where the textbook description reads, "Troublesome bleeding may ensue."

422. Today's pearl is tomorrow's fecalith.

423. Everyone is *not* trying to kill your patient.

424. There are just some things that will not heal, without bright lights and cold, sharp steel.

425. A calculated risk is when the surgeon does the calculating and the patient takes the risk.

426. You know the patient is in trouble when you start hearing vials popping at the head of the table.

427. There are old surgeons and bold surgeons, but few old, bold surgeons.

428. Be gentle when operating—imagine the noise if every cell could scream.

429. There is always more disease in the OR than there is in the angiography suite.

430. Remember that surgery is really about treating the patient, not just about offering a procedure.

431. There are fewer patients with too much disease than there are doctors with too little judgment.

432. When the number of redo procedures equals the number of primary operations, something is amiss.

433. In the OR, "truth" is defined as the opinion of the senior surgeon.

434. A medical curse:
May all your diseases be interesting.

435. A surgical curse:
May your operation be reportable.

436. What separates great surgeons from good surgeons is their postoperative care.

437. When plan A fails, make sure plan B is not the same as plan A.

438. It's OK not to know something as long as you know where to look it up or where to find someone who does know.

439. In most things surgical, the enemy of good is better.

440. A chance to cut is a chance to cure.

441. Placing the Foley catheter on suction is not an appropriate treatment for low urine output.

442. Don't hesitate to irrigate freely in contaminated cases. The solution to pollution is *dilution!*

443. When addressing problems in the OR, make sure your instruction is educational rather than punitive.

444. If things aren't going well, don't blame the instruments—that's a sign of a true amateur.

445. Reoperate selectively; if surgery didn't solve the problem the first time, a second procedure may not prove any better.

446. A smart surgeon knows he or she would rather be lucky than good.

447. Never operate against your better judgment.

448. Surgeons who exalt their cases shall be humbled.

449. Pride goeth before a bleeder.

450. It is the secret desire of every surgeon to leave this world with his or her name attached to an instrument or a procedure.

451. True vasculopaths have the equivalent of cancer of the blood vessels.

452. Remember that it is generally easier to *stay* out of trouble than it is to get out of trouble.

453. Don't worry about being fast, worry about being efficient.

454. There are more flavors of atherosclerotic disease than there are of Baskin-Robbins ice cream.

455. Just because an order is written doesn't mean that the job is done.

456. Poor surgeons need good anesthesiologists, excellent surgeons deserve them.

457. Don't excuse yourself for getting a patient in trouble, even if you are brilliant in getting the patient out.

458. After some minimally invasive procedures, the patient goes to recovery and the surgeon goes to intensive care.

459. One of the greatest rewards of private practice is that you can put the stitches *any damn place you want!*

Life's Lessons

". . . It is a wise man who can learn about one thing from another."

Plotinus

"All experience is an arch, to build upon."

Henry Brooks Adams

460. Your percentage of body fat and moral fiber should never approximate each other.

461. In surgery, chance definitely favors the prepared mind—the more prepared, the less the chance.

462. Go fast when you can so you may go slow when you must.

463. People will forget how quickly you did an operation; they will remember how *well* you did it!

464. There is no such thing as a courageous surgeon—it is the patient who bears the risk.

465. Never assume that just because something seems impossible, it couldn't happen.

466. If you find yourself first dialing "9" on your home phone, take a few days off.

467. The urologist's prayer—"Oh Lord, if I have to die, don't take me through my bladder."

468. If you operate for pain, you get pain.

469. Don't get a "vanity" license plate.

470. Keep a stash of chocolate candy in your desk drawer; it can get you through the last case of the day.

471. Surgeons who don't examine their mistakes are destined to repeat them.

472. Keep in mind the "3 As" of successful practice:
Be *A*ble.
Be *A*ffable.
Be *A*vailable.

473. It is forgivable to stop teaching but not to stop learning.

474. Purchase a good disability policy; a freak "minor" accident can end a career.

475. Take your family on a vacation that is not associated with a meeting or a conference.

476. Know how to use a personal computer for more than games and e-mail.

477. It is impossible not to take a lawsuit personally.

478. Don't smoke.

479. Avoid the pursuit of meaningless midlife trophies.

480. Complain infrequently—you knew the job was tough when you took it.

481. Never do something in the OR just to see if you can.

482. Don't shoot the messengers, unless, of course, they also happen to be the perpetrators.

483. More important than having a great idea is *recognizing* a great idea.

484. Remember that for medicolegal purposes, if it's not in the chart, it didn't occur.

485. In very difficult situations, never underestimate the power of persistence.

486. Avoid being a "hired gun" for plaintiff attorneys in malpractice litigation.

487. If a litigious individual tells you, "It's not the money," be assured *it's the money!*

488. Don't forget that very bad outcomes can occur even in the hands of very good surgeons.

489. Most surgery is 70% *competence* and 30% *confidence.*

490. Unfortunately, you can't look at the world through 3.5× glasses.

491. If you ever find yourself uttering the term "culprit lesion" during cardiac surgery, seek counseling from a surgical colleague immediately.

492. Practice long enough and you will probably
see everything.

493. Cut your own lawn; it is very therapeutic.

494. Even on your last day of practice there will be
something new to learn.

495. Don't try to be all things to all people.

496. You cannot outrun statistics.

497. Realize early on that you cannot make enough money to compensate for an unhappy home.

498. The pioneering surgeons were simply not mortals.

499. It is possible to be skeptical without being cynical.

500. Confidence is essential; arrogance
is deadly.

501. Take your work seriously, yourself less so.

502. About the time you get it all figured out, it is time to retire.

503. The better you are, the luckier you get.

504. Don't take journals with you on vacations.

505. Don't skip your religious obligations to make rounds.

506. Surprise your children by picking them up at school once in a while.

507. It is good to learn from your mistakes but better to learn from someone else's.

508. Find a middle ground between being a missionary and being a mercenary.

509. Give yourself a break now and then.

510. If your number of ex-spouses exceeds your number of ex-partners, you have a serious problem.

511. Learn to trust your instincts.

512. There is no substitute for experience.

513. Don't behave badly just because you can.

514. You can't possibly read enough.

515. Never let your mouth write checks your *curriculum vitae* can't cash.

516. In the long run, your accomplishments as a parent or a spouse will far outweigh *anything* you do in the OR.

517. Be more impressed by how much you have to learn than by how much you know.

518. Unrelenting stress *will* ultimately kill you.

519. If you love your work but hate your job, it might be time to look elsewhere.

520. Life is short—Buy a fast computer.

521. Never own a pager that is smarter than you are.

522. *Illegitimi non carborundum*—Don't let the bastards wear you down.

523. Don't ever let being a *surgeon* get in the way of being a *doctor*.

524. A toast to your colleagues: "May you never be a great case."

525. Strive not to measure your worth by your W-2.

526. Busy surgeons are happy surgeons.

527. It is easy to become cocky; it is hard to stay that way.

528. Surgeons tend to get along better because they see each other in their underwear on a regular basis.

529. An arrogant attitude and a limited knowledge base is a most dangerous combination.

530. In surgery, success is ultimately in the details.

531. The *Positions Wanted* sections are full of "irreplaceable" surgeons.

532. Surgeons are like pianists; there are technicians and there are artists.

533. There is no clinical situation that cannot be compared to baseball.

534. Be famous at home, first.

535. The day you think it is really all *you*—it is time to *QUIT!*

Notes